"The Idea is to Die Young"

~ English anthropologis

Sugar Free Budget Cooking for One

Sugar Free Supper Recipes to Help Control Diabetes & Lose Weight

Recipes for a Sugar Free Life

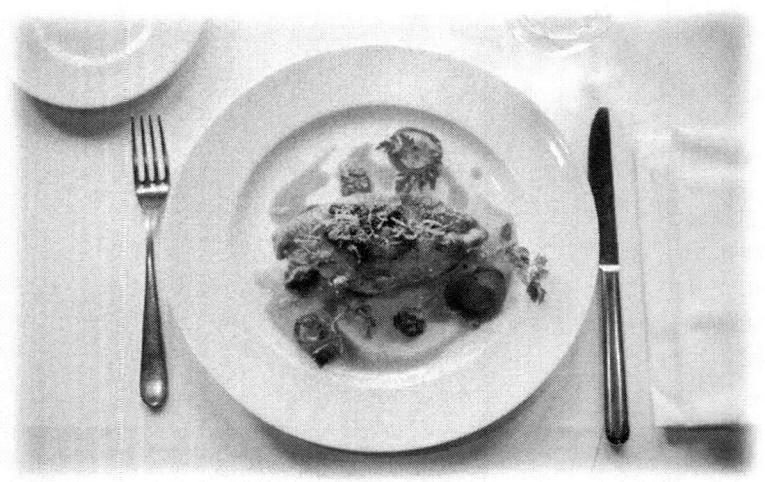

DISCLAIMER

All information in the book is for general information purposes only.

The author has used her best efforts in preparing this information and makes no representations or warranties with respect to the accuracy, applicability or completeness of the material contained within.

Furthermore, the author takes no responsibility for any errors, omissions or inaccuracies in this document. The author disclaims any implied or expressed warranties or fitness for any particular purpose.

The author shall in no event be held liable for losses or damages whatsoever. The author assumes no responsibility or liability for any consequences resulting directly or indirectly from any action or lack of action that you take based on the information in this document.

Use of the publication and recipes therein is at your own risk.

Reproduction or translation of any part of this publication by any means, electronic or mechanical, without the permission of the author, is both forbidden and illegal. You are not permitted to share, sell, and trade or give away this document and it is for your own personal use only, unless stated otherwise.

By using any of the recipes in this publication, you agree that you have read the disclaimer and agree with all the terms.

The reader assumes full risk and responsibility for all actions taken as a result of the information contained within this book and the author will not be held responsible for any loss or damage, whether consequential, incidental, or otherwise that may result from the information presented in this book.

The author has relied on her own experiences when compiling this book and each recipe is tried and tested in her own kitchen.

Contents

Introduction	6
Tasty Tuna Burgers	10
Pork Chop with Apple and Mustard	12
Supreme Omelet and Cheese	14
Chicken with Leek Sauce	15
Vegetable Rice and Pesto Bowl	16
Italian Style Pork Steak	18
Shrimp Stuffed Avocado	19
Easy Chicken and Coconut Curry	20
Parsnip and Coconut Soup	22
Zucchini and Fish Fritter	23
Simple Chicken Casserole	24
Easy Tomato Soup	25
Crispy Herby Chicken	26
Spicy Salmon with Caramelized Onion	28
Pork Schnitzel	30
Parmesan Chicken Goujons	32
Mediterranean Style Baked Eggs	34
Creamy White Wine Chicken	36
Sundried Tomato and Scallion Stuffed Zucchini	38
Tuna and Tomato Bake	40
Sweet Potato and Green Bean Curry	42
Smoky Bacon and Roast Pepper Warm Salad	44
Sweet Chili Butternut Squash and Sweet Potato Soup	46
Chinese Crab Stick Mushroom and Scallion Soup	47
Chicken Rolls	48
Individual Crustless Quiche	50
Beetroot Burgers	52
Leek Lasagne	54
Meatloaf Muffin	56
Roasted Cauliflower Salad	58
Mushroom Risotto	60
Vegetable Medley Italian Style	62
Zucchini and Cheese Frittata	64
Cauliflower Rice Chicken Stir Fry	66
Eggs in Bacon Baskets	68
Garlic and Lemon Beef Tips	70
Baked Vegetable Stuffed Eggplant	72
Baked Fish in Foil	74
Speedy Chicken Chili	76
Barbeque Chicken	78

Sweet Potato and Tuna Burgers	80
Bacon and Chickpea Chunky Soup	82
Rocket and Avocado Salad	84
Mediterranean Sunday Brunch	85
Sautéed Shrimp Fennel and Tomatoes	86
Harissa Chicken with Quinoa	87
Spanish Mackerel	88
Spiced Yogurt Chicken	90
Butternut Squash and Goats Cheese Bake	91
Peppered Beef with Sweet Potato Cakes	92
Lamb with Pea and Rosemary Mash	93
Thank You	94
Measurements and Conversions	95

Introduction

When I moved to my current address 18 months ago I had to join a new Doctors practice. I went for the initial tests they always give you in UK; blood tests, height, weight etc. and having asthma, I had to go to the asthma clinic for a checkup. Everything was fine as far as I knew because I didn't hear anything to the contrary; I assumed they would call if anything was not as it should be.

I am very rarely ill and easily manage the asthma with inhalers so avoid going to the Doctors for anything unless I absolutely have to. When I got a letter to say my annual asthma review was due, I made the appointment (otherwise they would stop the repeat prescription for the inhalers…).

I attended the clinic and a simple remark from the asthma nurse gave me quite a shock. She said it was on my records that she had to remind me to make an appointment for a fasting glucose test. When I asked why, she told me the last one 12 months previously was in the pre-diabetic range – 7.3. I had no idea what that meant but made the appointment and went home to do a bit of research.

I did have gestational diabetes when expecting the second of my five sons but it disappeared once I was delivered. That was nearly 40 years ago so I never gave it another thought.

Before I went for the second fasting blood test I had been trying to lose a bit of weight so had been eating a bit healthier than normal; not as many sugary desserts or bars of chocolate. The result showed that the level had dropped to 6.5.

A relief but definitely an eye opener. I certainly didn't want to be one of the thousands of people who are diagnosed each year with diabetes so decided to do something about it.

I am a firm believer in the Universe providing the answer to our problems – if we take the time to look and listen. This is how I came across the concept of **sugar free living**.

I was driving into town one day shortly after the second fasting glucose test and was listening to the radio while I was sitting in the usual traffic jam. I caught a conversation between Dr. Michael Mosley and Chris Evans on BBC Radio 2 about sugar free living. It caught my imagination so when I got home I bought the book, '**The 8 Week Blood Sugar Diet**' by Dr. Michael Mosley. It was a revelation and answered a lot of questions I had about diabetes and diet. I did consider following the weight loss program included in the book but decided it was a bit too restrictive for me but was convinced that living as sugar free as possible could help.

The funny thing is, once I had got the 'bit between my teeth' about this new way of living, I began to notice lots of other information beginning to appear. The national news programs were full of a volte-face about the low-fat approach to dieting, saying that since the UK Government began to recommend low fat diets, obesity has risen four-fold possibly due to the amount of sugar used to improve the taste of low or 0% fat foods. But the jury is still out on that. The argument continues...

However, I welcome the fact that, using the sugar free approach as outlined by Dr. Mosley, I can eat a reasonable amount of cheese, butter, oil and nuts without feeling guilty while reducing the chance of becoming diabetic. Obviously, you must use some common sense and not overdo the fat content in your diet.

I bought a water filter jug and have been surprised by the difference in the *smell* of the water. I now only use filtered water for everything I consume; hot drinks, cold drinks and even water for cooking. I don't know if there are any health benefits but just the fact that the tap water smells of chemicals is enough to persuade me to change.

Previously I have tried to cut down on processed food, reasoning that nature has provided us with good nutritious food from vegetables, fruit, meat and dairy so why would it be beneficial for us to eat food that has had stuff added, removed or that has been tinkered with?

So, after reading Dr. Mosley's book from cover to cover – then reading it again, I decided to try and live my life sugar free, **eating only meals that I have prepared at home using fresh ingredients**. No ready meals or processed food.

I have looked all over for affordable sugar free recipes for **one person** but most books and websites have recipes for two or four people.

So, to make things easier and more affordable for those of us that need sugar free recipes for just one person I have devised these 'Budget Cooking for One ~ Sugar Free Supper Recipes to Help Control Diabetes and Lose Weight'.

Not all of the recipes are completely sugar free because a lot of foods contain naturally occurring sugars – do your own research if you are at all unsure about the sugar content of any ingredient. For instance, I was stunned to discover just how much sugar is in a small pot of zero fat natural yoghurt...

Even without realizing it most of us are eating between **22 and 37 teaspoons of sugar a day**, a lot of it being hidden in processed foods.

So please check the labels of anything you buy to make sure there is no hidden sugar – any ingredient ending in '**ose**' is usually sugar.

I really hope this book will inspire you to take control of your own health by eating natural food as it was intended. No preservatives, just fresh ingredients. To be honest, I've found it doesn't take up much time to cook from scratch and hope you will give it a go too.

Don't forget, no-one else can decide what we put into our body so it's up to all of us to TAKE CONTROL and only eat and drink stuff that we know is natural and has not been messed with.

Let's get to the recipes...

Tasty Tuna Burgers

This recipe will make 4 Tuna Burgers. I usually freeze three of them individually and take one out of the freezer before I go to work so I have a quick dinner when I get home.

Ingredients

1 can of tuna, drained
½ cup wheat bran
½ cup diced celery
1 small chopped onion
1 egg
2 tbsp tomato puree
1 tsp lemon juice
Small amount of oil

Method

Put the oil in a skillet (frying pan) and fry the celery for a minute or two. Add the onion and fry for a further two minutes. Tip onto kitchen paper and leave to go cold.

Mix all the ingredients together then form into 4 patties. Place on lightly greased baking tray and cook in the oven for 20-25 minutes or until cooked through.

Served with a green salad, it is a delicious and filling meal.

Note: If you are freezing the Tuna Burgers allow to go cold before wrapping separately and putting in freezer.

Notes:

Pork Chop with Apples and Mustard

This delicious dish takes less than 30 minutes to make at home. It tastes incredible and the sauce adds an amazing flavor to the pork.

Ingredients

1 apple
1 tbsp olive oil
1 pork chop
2 scallions (spring onions)
2 tbsp cream
1 tsp mustard (more if you like mustard)
¼ tsp dried thyme
Selection of vegetables of your choice
Seasoning to taste

Method

Heat oven to 300°.

Chop your chosen vegetables (I used cherry tomatoes, zucchini (courgette), onion and thinly sliced peppers) and coat in half of the oil. Season with salt and pepper then roast in the oven for around 20 minutes.

Meanwhile heat the rest of the olive oil in the frying pan, chop the scallions and cook for 2 minutes then add the pork chop and fry for 2 minutes each side. Season to taste.

Wash and core the apple, then chop into chunks (no need to peel unless you want to).

Add the apple chunks and turn the heat down. Cook for around 3 minutes, stirring the ingredients occasionally.

Put the cream, mustard and thyme into a small bowl and mix together.

Put the mixture in the pan with the apples and pork chop and stir together. Simmer the ingredients over low heat for another 3 minutes or until pork is cooked.

Serve immediately with the roasted vegetables.

Supreme Omelet with Cheese

Ingredients

2 eggs
1 scallion (spring onion)
1 pepper
Large handful spinach
3-4 cherry tomatoes - quartered
1 cup shredded cheese
Tbsp. water
Seasoning to taste
Butter

Method

Put butter in a skillet over a medium heat. Finely chop scallion and pepper then add to skillet and sauté for 2 minutes before adding the tomatoes. Sauté for a further 2 minutes then add the spinach.

Meanwhile, whisk eggs, water and seasoning together. Pour over the vegetables just as the spinach has wilted and cook until the egg just begins to set.

Sprinkle with the shredded cheese, fold over then slide onto your serving plate.

Add a large salad or some seasonal vegetables and enjoy.

Note: The trick to the perfect omelet is NOT to OVERCOOK it, no-one likes rubber eggs so remove from the heat while the top is still soft.

Chicken with Leek Sauce

This is a lovely chicken dish and is quick and easy to prepare.

Ingredients

1 boneless chicken breast
1 large leek
1 tbsp butter
1 clove garlic
1 tsp. wholegrain mustard
Small glass dry white wine
1 tbsp. cream

Method

Peel and crush the garlic. Trim leeks and cut into 1cm slices.

Melt the butter in a pan and add the garlic and chicken. Fry the chicken on both sides until it is a nice golden brown. Stir in the leeks, mustard and wine.

Bring the mixture to the boil adding a little water if necessary. Reduce the heat, cover and simmer for around 20 minutes or until the chicken is cooked through.

Stir the cream into the pan. Taste and season to your liking. Serve immediately with some sweet potato mash.

Note: When using wine in cooking, only use wine that you would drink yourself. If you wouldn't drink a glass of it yourself, it would not improve in any dish.

Vegetable, Rice and Pesto Bowl

This is a very tasty way to use up any leftover vegetables that you have sitting in your fridge. You could also add any leftover cold meat to the salad if you like. This salad is a great picnic dish or as an accompaniment to a steak. Great for a lunchbox too. The vegetables listed below are simply suggestions; use whatever you have available.

Ingredients

1 cup whole grain rice
Cherry tomatoes
Red pepper
Green pepper
Spring onions
Few slices of cucumber

For the dressing:
1 clove garlic
Tbsp. pesto
Tbsp. white wine vinegar
2 tbsp. good olive oil
Seasoning

Method

Rinse the rice and cook using the 2 to 1 method (2 parts water to 1 part rice). Drain the rice and rinse under cold running water. Transfer to your chosen serving bowl.

Chop your vegetables into very small dice. Mix into the rice thoroughly.

Peel and crush the clove of garlic. Add the garlic to the pesto, white wine vinegar and olive oil. Whisk until well combined. Drizzle the dressing over the rice salad and toss. Serve immediately.

Note: If you are taking this in a lunchbox to work, put the dressing in a separate container and add just before eating.

Italian Style Pork Steak

Pork is a very reasonably price meat and can be very tasty if not overcooked. This recipe is simple to make and adds a bit of an Italian flavor to your meal for a change.

Ingredients

1 lean pork steak
1 tbsp. oil
1 small onion
1 or 2 cloves garlic
1 tbsp. chopped fresh rosemary
1 tsp. grated lemon zest
1 tbsp. finely chopped oregano
½ cup chicken stock
½ can chopped tomatoes
Seasoning

Method

Heat the oil in a frying pan and cook pork steak for about 2 minutes on each side or until nicely browned. Remove from pan.

Peel and finely chop the onion and, using the same pan, cook until soft and transparent. Add a little more oil if needed. Peel and crush the garlic and add to the onions with the chopped rosemary, oregano and lemon zest. Cook for a further minute. Add the stock and tomatoes, bring to the boil.

Reduce the heat and return the pork steak to the pan. Simmer over a low heat for 10-12 minutes or until the pork steak is cooked through and the sauce is slightly thickened.

Remove from the heat, taste and season to your liking.

Shrimp Stuffed Avocado

Ingredients

1 avocado
1 cup cooked shrimps
2 cloves garlic
½ tbsp extra virgin olive oil
½ cup parsley
½ tbsp lemon juice
Chili powder to taste
Sea salt
Pepper

Method

Cut the avocado in half and remove the pit. Finely chop the parsley.

Scrape out the avocado flesh and keep the shell. Chop the avocado flesh and place in a large bowl. Crush the garlic and add to the bowl.

Add the cooked shrimps, chopped parsley, extra virgin olive oil, lemon juice and chili powder. Stir gently until well combined. Taste and season.

Take the avocado shells and using a spoon, fill them with the mixture from the bowl. Serve with a green salad.

Easy Chicken and Coconut Curry

The joy of cooking a curry for yourself is you are free to experiment with the spices. For example, I don't like a lot of ginger or chili so I only add a tiny bit of each for this dish but I would add a bit more cilantro (coriander) because I love it.

Ingredients

½ can coconut milk (the other half can be used for Parsnip and Coconut Soup on next page)
Small bunch cilantro (coriander)
2 large garlic cloves
Small piece fresh root ginger
1 green chili
1 tbsp. olive oil
2-3 skinless chicken thighs or drumsticks
1 small onion, finely chopped
Small piece of cinnamon stick or 1 tsp cinnamon powder
1 tsp cumin powder
1 tsp cilantro powder
1 tsp Garam masala

Method

Blend the coconut milk and cilantro in a food processor, then tip out and set aside. Put the garlic, ginger and chili into the food processor, and blend with enough water to make a paste.

Heat the oil in a large pan. Brown the chicken well then remove. Add the chopped onion and cinnamon and fry until onion is golden. Add the chili paste to the pan and cook until most of the liquid has evaporated.

Stir in the powdered spices plus the coconut milk and cilantro paste then return the chicken to the pan. Bring to a boil, cover and cook for 30-40 minutes, remove the lid halfway through to thicken the sauce.

Check the chicken is cooked, season to taste adding a splash of water if the sauce has thickened too much.

Serve with wholegrain rice garnished with a few cilantro leaves.

Parsnip and Coconut Soup

This soup is a great standby to have in the fridge for when you need a quick supper.

Ingredients

3 parsnips
1 small white onion
1 clove garic
½ can of coconut milk
Chives for garnish (optional)
Seasoning

Method

Peel and chop the parsnips and onion into small chunks. Boil in lightly salted water until soft. Drain well. Put the parsnips and onion into a blender along with the crushed garlic adding coconut milk a little at a time until you get your preferred consistency. Blend until smooth.

Return to pan and reheat. Garnish with finely chopped chives (if using) and serve with a chunk of wholegrain bread.

Zucchini and Fish Fritters

Ingredients

1 egg
Piece of firm fish – your choice (I use cod)
½ zucchini (courgette) grated
½ sweet potato grated
Handful grated cheese (optional)
Seasoning
1 tbsp. olive oil
Small knob of butter

Method

Cut the fish into small, bite sized pieces. Whisk the egg well and add the fish, grated zucchini, grated sweet potato, grated cheese (if used) and salt and pepper to taste. Mix until well combined.

Heat the olive oil in a frying pan. Drop spoonfuls of the mixture into the pan and cook for around 4 minutes on each side. Towards the end of cooking, add the butter and spoon over the fritters to glaze.

These are delicious served with a crisp green salad.

Simple Chicken Casserole

This casserole has been a great standby for when unexpected guests arrive, I simply increased the recipe according to the number of guests. But it is just as simple to make for one person.

Ingredients

1 chicken fillet
1 small red onion
3 large mushrooms
½ can plum tomatoes (the other half can be used to make Easy Tomato Soup on next page)
1 tsp dried mixed herbs
1 tbsp olive oil
Salt and pepper

Method

Heat the olive oil in a frying pan. Chop the onion and add to the pan. Stir-fry until golden.

Add the chicken fillet to the pan and brown on both sides.

Thinly slice the mushrooms and add these along with the dried herbs to the pan. Stir-fry until golden.

Chop the tomatoes then add to the pan, bring to a gentle simmer and allow to cook until the chicken is cooked through, approximately 15 minutes. If the pan starts to dry out add some cold water.

Taste and season to your liking. Serve with lots of green vegetables.

Easy Tomato Soup

Ingredients

½ can plum tomatoes
4 fresh ripe tomatoes
1 small onion
1 clove garlic
1 carrot
1 chicken or vegetable stock cube
Oil

Method

Chop the onion and grate the carrot and garlic. Heat the oil in a pan and add the vegetables and garlic. Cook over a medium heat for about 3 minutes.

Dissolve the stock cube in about 2 cups of water and add to the pan along with the tinned and fresh tomatoes. Bring to the boil stirring well then reduce heat and simmer for around 7-10 minutes.

Using a blender (a stick type will do the job), blend until smooth. You could add a few basil leaves before blending for an extra flavor hit.

Reheat and add a swirl of cream before serving.

Note: For a more substantial meal, add some cooked pasta shells before reheating.

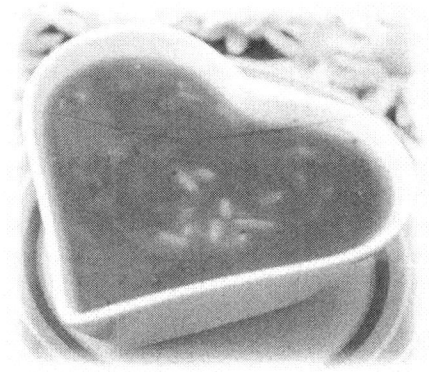

Crispy Herby Chicken

A good dish to prepare and leave to marinate before you go to work ready to cook for dinner.

Ingredients

2 chicken thighs or 1 breast with skin on
Extra-virgin olive oil as needed
½ tbsp. chopped fresh rosemary
1 tsp chopped fresh oregano
½ tsp dried thyme (or 1 tsp fresh thyme)
½ tsp garlic powder
Salt and pepper to taste

Method

Preheat the oven to 375°F. Place chicken into an oven proof baking dish.

Mix rosemary, oregano, thyme, garlic powder, salt and pepper together in a bowl. At this stage you could add any other herbs or spices you want, like chili flakes to give the dish a little kick. Add oil until you achieve a thin paste. Pour over chicken and shake the baking dish to coat well.
Cover anc leave in refrigerator to marinate for a couple of hours.

Cover with foil and bake for around 25-35 minutes (or until chicken is cooked through) in the preheated oven. Remove the foil and return to the oven uncovered for the last 5 minutes. Baste regularly for extra crispness.

Serve immediately with your choice of vegetables.

Notes:

Spicy Salmon with Caramelized Onions

Although the ingredient list looks long, it is mainly seasonings for the salmon fillet. You can try any mix of your preferred herbs and spices for the rub. The fun of these type of dishes is the experimentation to get a mix you like.

Ingredients

1 salmon fillet
1 – 2 tbsp. chopped onion
½ teaspoon ground black pepper
½ tsp paprika
1 tsp balsamic vinegar
¼ tsp cayenne pepper
1 tsp minced garlic or garlic powder
1 tsp Dijon mustard
½ tsp onion powder
¼ tsp salt
1 tbsp. olive oil

Method

Combine the black pepper, paprika, cayenne pepper, minced garlic, Dijon mustard, onion powder, and salt in a small bowl. Stir in ½ tbsp. of olive oil to make a paste. Spread the paste all over the salmon fillets, and set aside to marinate at room temperature for around 30 - 45 minutes. You could even prepare this in the morning before work and leave to marinate until you come home for a quick and tasty supper.

Heat the remaining olive oil in a small pan over medium heat. Add the onion, and cook until tender and golden brown, about 8 minutes then stir in the balsamic vinegar.

Heat a separate non-stick skillet over medium-high heat and cook the salmon fillet skin side down until skin is crisp then turn and cook until the fillet is no longer translucent in the center, about 4 minutes per side. Pour the browned onions and olive oil over the salmon fillet and serve with your choice of vegetables.

Pork Schnitzel

I will assume for this recipe that you are making schnitzel for one meal. However, the oatmeal, egg and flour will coat a couple of pork steaks so I usually make extra to use up the oatmeal mixture. They freeze really well and don't take long to defrost for a quick and easy meal.

Ingredients

1 or 2 pork steaks
½ cup all-purpose white flour
½ cup fine oatmeal
1 egg
1 tsp paprika
½ tbsp. finely chopped chives
1 tsp garlic powder
Salt and pepper to taste

Method

Bash the pork between 2 sheets of plastic wrap (cling film) with meat mallet or, if you don't have one, the bottom of a saucepan or a rolling pin, until the meat is about ¼ inch thick.

Arrange 3 shallow bowls or pie plates with the following; flour seasoned with salt and pepper in the first, beaten egg in the second, and oatmeal mixed with garlic powder, chives and paprika in the third.

Cover pork slices first in flour, dip in beaten egg and finally coat in the oatmeal mixture. At this stage you can wrap and freeze any you are not using immediately.

Heat a skillet over medium heat. Add 1 tbsp. butter and ½ tbsp. olive oil. When oil is hot, add pork. Cook until golden brown on each side, about 1 to 2 minutes per side. Add a little more butter to the pan if it becomes too dry during cooking.

Remove schnitzel from pan. Transfer to paper towel to drain. Keep warm until ready to serve.

Goes really well with green vegetables or a large salad.

Note: Try adding different herbs and spices to the oatmeal to find the mix that you like best. You could substitute chicken breast for the pork to make your schnitzel if you prefer – the method is the same.

Parmesan Chicken Goujons

Children love these homemade chicken goujons (a 'goujon' is a small strip of fish or chicken, coated in crumbs), they are the healthy alternative to the ones you can buy from the takeaway. So, although these are delicious for supper dish, they are quick and easy to make when children are visiting.

Ingredients

½ cup fine oatmeal
1 boneless, skinless chicken breast
1 egg
2 tbsp. grated Parmesan cheese
1 tsp dried oregano
salt and pepper
1 tbsp. oil
Butter

Method

Cut chicken lengthwise into strips about 1 inch thick.

Break egg into shallow dish; using fork, beat well. In another shallow dish, stir together oatmeal, Parmesan cheese, oregano, salt and pepper.

Dip chicken strips into egg, letting excess drip off; dip in crumb mixture, turning to coat all sides.

Arrange on a greased baking sheet; drizzle with butter. Bake in preheated oven 425°F until golden, crispy and no longer pink inside, about 10 -15 minutes.

Serve with a side salad and a small dish of garlic mayonnaise (or just simple mayonnaise if you prefer).

Note: You could also use any type of firm fish instead of chicken for this recipe.

Mediterranean-Style Baked Eggs

These are great for a light meal and really simple to make. The ingredient list is simply a suggestion and can be altered to your own preference – the beauty of cooking for one.

Ingredients

2 eggs
1 tbsp. chopped olives, black or green, your choice
1 tbsp. diced tomatoes
1 tbsp. chopped fresh spinach
1 tbsp. feta cheese
1 tbsp. chopped basil
Salt and pepper

Method

Preheat the oven to 350^0F

In a mixing bowl, whisk the eggs then add all the ingredients and stir until thoroughly combined.

Spray 2 compartments of a muffin tray, or 2 oven-proof ramekins with non-stick cooking spray

Pour the mixture in each of the two compartments (or ramekins). Bake for around 10 minutes or until set and golden brown.

Using a rubber spatula, ease the eggs out of their compartments to a plate.

Serve with a crisp green salad.

Note: With this recipe you can add almost any ingredient you prefer. For example, if you don't like olives you could add a slice of cooked bacon chopped into small cubes.
The vegetables can be exchanged for whatever you prefer. Your imagination is your best friend…

Creamy White Wine Chicken

This baked chicken breast sits on a bed of leeks and covered with a creamy white wine sauce – delicious.

Ingredients

1 large chicken breast
1 clove garlic
1 tbsp. chopped parsley
1 tbsp. olive oil
1 small leek
1 tsp cornstarch
2 tbsp. white wine
2 tbsp. cream
2 tbsp. cold water
Salt and pepper

Method

Preheat the oven to 425°F.

Mix minced garlic, parsley and 2 teaspoons of the oil in a small bowl.

Cut around 4 slits along the top of the chicken breast then rub the herb mixture all over especially over the cuts to make sure the mixture flavors the meat.

Spread the sliced leek loosely over the base of a small ovenproof dish – not too big or the sauce will burn. Add the remaining oil and toss the leeks to coat.

Place the chicken on top, season and bake for around 10 minutes. While the chicken is cooking, mix the cornstarch and wine until smooth and whisk in the cream and water.

Take the chicken out of the oven and pour the sauce over. Return to the oven for 10 – 15 minutes or until the chicken is cooked through.

Transfer the chicken to a serving plate and stir the leeks and cream sauce then pour over chicken.

This dish is really nice with wholegrain wild rice.

Sun-dried Tomato and Scallion Stuffed Zucchini

This appetizing, vegetarian dish makes a delicious lunch served with a light salad.

Ingredients

1 large zucchini (courgette)
3 or 4 pieces of sun-dried tomatoes in oil (well drained and chopped)
2 scallions (spring onions)
1 egg
½ teaspoon dried mixed herbs
1 tbsp low fat cream cheese
1 tbsp shredded cheese (optional)
Salt and pepper to taste

Method

Put the whole zucchini in a pan of salted boiling water, and cook for 5 minutes.

Remove zucchini from pan, and cut in half length ways. Scoop out ¾ of the flesh, squeeze out excess juice and chop.

Cover zucchini shell in aluminum foil, and put in oven on very low heat to keep warm.

In a bowl, mix together eggs, cream cheese, sun-dried tomatoes, chopped scallions, mixed herbs, zucchini flesh, and salt and pepper to taste. Mix well with fork.

Heat the egg mixture in a non-stick pan on a low heat until it is lightly firmed.

Remove the zucchini from oven and spoon the egg mixture into the shells. Sprinkle with shredded cheese (if using) and place under a hot grill until cheese is melted.

Note: Eggplant (aubergine) can be used instead of zucchini for this recipe.

Tuna and Tomato Bake

This is a great 'stand by' dish for when you have surprise visitors as nearly everyone I know has a tin of tuna and a tin of tomatoes in the back of the cupboard. This recipe makes enough for two servings so I usually make it up then freeze one portion for another day.

Ingredients

1 tin Tuna in spring water
1 tin tomatoes
2 fresh tomatoes
1 medium onion
1 tbsp tomato puree
2 cups Orzo pasta (Orzo, also risoni, is a form of short-cut pasta, shaped like a large grain of rice)
1 tsp dried oregano
½ tsp chili flakes (optional)
1 clove garlic
Shredded cheese
Oil
Salt and pepper

Method

Finely chop the onion and garlic then fry in oil until softened. Add the tin of tomatoes stirring well to break up them up.

Add oregano and chili flakes. Cook for a couple of minutes over a medium heat.

Add the whole tin of tuna (no need to drain) and stir in. Chop the fresh tomatoes and add those to the pan along with the tomato puree, stir well trying not to break up the tuna too much.

Bring back to boil then add the orzo. Reduce heat to low and cook until orzo is soft. If the sauce gets too thick add more water. Add salt and pepper to taste.

Once the orzo is cooked to your liking – I like mine quite soft, divide between two ovenproof dishes then sprinkle with cheese. Place under grill until cheese is golden brown.

Note: If you are freezing one portion you can put it in a freezer bag then, when you want to use it, thaw it thoroughly. Warm through in a pan then transfer to ovenproof dish, add cheese then grill as before.

Sweet Potato and Green Bean Curry

Curries are a tasty treat, but can be very high in fat content. This quick and easy recipe is a delicious, healthy alternative and is packed with flavor.

Ingredients

1 large sweet potato (peeled and chopped into medium chunks)
1 handful of green beans (cut in half)
½ onion (peeled and diced)
2 cloves garlic (finely chopped)
2 tbsp cream cheese
1 tbsp oil
2 tbsp milk (you could use coconut milk if you like)
1 tbsp curry paste (as mild or hot as you like)
Salt and pepper to taste

Method

Boil sweet potato chunks in salted water until tender. Throw the green beans in for the last five minutes. Drain the vegetables and keep warm

Put garlic, onion and oil in a bowl and mix well.

Heat a pan to a medium heat, add garlic and onions and cook until slightly golden. Add curry paste to pan and stir through.

Turn down to a low heat, and add cream cheese, milk and the vegetables to the curry mixture. Cook for around 5 minutes until piping hot. Season to taste.

Serve in a warmed dish with boiled wholegrain rice.

Notes:

Smoky Bacon and Roast Pepper Warm Salad

This rich, smoky warm salad makes a sumptuous evening meal, served with nothing more than plenty of freshly milled black pepper.

Ingredients

2 slices of lean smoked bacon
1 medium red pepper
4 cherry tomatoes
2 cloves garlic (peeled and sliced)
½ teaspoon oregano
½ teaspoon dried basil
2 teaspoons smoked paprika
Parmesan shavings
1 tbsp olive oil
Salt and pepper to taste
Salad Leaves

Method

Preheat oven to 450°F

Cut pepper in half and remove seeds and white flesh. Divide garlic between peppers.

Sprinkle peppers with oregano, dried basil, smoked paprika and seasoning.

Drizzle olive oil over the garlic inside the peppers. Roast for 15 minutes.

Remove from oven and add the cherry tomatoes to the peppers and roast for another 10-15 minutes.

Put the bacon in the oven in a separate oven dish for the last 10-15 minute until the bacon is cooked.

Remove stalks from peppers and chop the bacon into substantial pieces.

Arrange salad leaves on your serving dish, place your two halves of pepper on top then add the bacon. Sprinkle with the parmesan shavings.

Season to taste and serve immediately.

Sweet Chili, Butternut Squash and Sweet Potato Soup

A hearty, wholesome soup that makes a substantial lunch. Serve with a slice of granary bread.

Ingredients

¼ butternut squash (peeled and diced)
1 sweet potato (peeled and diced)
¾ pint of chicken stock
1 dessert spoon of sweet chili sauce
A good pinch of cumin
Salt and pepper to taste

Method

Put the butternut squash and sweet potato in a pan on the hob, and cover with chicken stock.

Bring the stock to the boil and reduce to simmer for ½ hour. Remove from heat and allow to cool.

Put the stock and vegetables in a blender, and blend until the consistency is thick and creamy

Put the soup in a clean pan, and add the sweet chili sauce and cumin, season to taste, and stir well.

Allow the soup to heat through without bringing it to the boil.

Serve in a warmed bowl.

Chinese Crab Stick, Mushroom and Scallion Soup

Chinese takeaways can be a real treat on a Friday night, but tend to be heavy in fat and MSG. This hearty soup delivers aromatic, oriental flavors that are kinder on your pocket and waistline. Quick and easy to make after a hard day at work.

Ingredients

5 crab sticks (shredded)
3 scallions (spring onions) (chopped)
6 mushrooms (sliced)
½ pint Chicken Stock
Pinch of white pepper
1 teaspoon of light soy sauce
½ teaspoon of sesame oil
2 cloves of garlic
½ inch fresh ginger peeled

Method

Peel cloves of garlic and ginger, and lightly crush to help release the flavors.

Add garlic and ginger to chicken stock, and bring to the boil. Reduce heat and allow stock to simmer for 10 minutes.

Remove garlic and ginger, and add sliced mushrooms and scallions. Simmer for another 5 minutes, and then add remaining ingredients. Simmer for another 2 minutes and serve in a warmed bowl.

Chicken Rolls

If you are looking for a simple meal but delicious in the same time, this recipe is for you. It's quick and easy and you can prepare the rolls in advance.

Ingredients

½ tbsp olive oil
¼ green bell pepper
¼ red bell pepper
½ onion
½ lb chicken fingers or 1 chicken breast cut into fingers
½ tbsp taco seasoning

Method

Preheat the oven to 375° F.

Slice the green and red bell peppers and onion. Place them in a saucepan and sauté in the olive oil over medium to high heat for around 5-7 minutes.

When the peppers are tender and the onion turns opaque, sprinkle some of the taco seasoning over them. If you don't have any you can use your favorite herb or spice combination. Your dish will be tasty either way.

Place the chicken fingers on a cutting board. Using a meat mallet or rolling pin, bash the fingers until they become thin and flat.

Use taco seasoning to sprinkle the surface of the chicken fingers.

Make small stacks of the sliced peppers and onion. Place a stack in the center of each chicken finger and roll up. Use a toothpick to fix the end of the chicken roll-up and sprinkle with more of the taco seasoning. At this point you can put them in the refrigerator to pop in the oven when you get home from work.

Bake the rolls in the preheated oven for 12 minutes or until chicken is cooked and slightly brown.

Serve immediately with a jacket sweet potato or a salad.

Individual Crustless Quiche

Ingredients

1 egg
1 tbsp. milk
1 cup finely chopped vegetable of your choice
1 slice ham finely chopped
½ cup shredded cheese

Method

Preheat oven to 350°F.

Place egg and milk into a bowl and whisk together.

Stir in the chopped vegetables and ham.

Line a muffin tin with paper cases or grease the tin if not using cases.

Fill each case with the mixture then sprinkle with grated cheese.

Bake in oven until egg mixture is almost set with a very slight wobble in the middle.

Remove from oven and leave to cool before removing from tin.

Delicious either hot or cold.

Note: These are great to add to a lunchbox with a crisp salad or easy to pack to take on a picnic. Most children love these.

Beetroot Burgers

Ingredients

1lb of vac packed beetroot (mine was 4 beets-leaving one in the pack) chopped
1 tin of drained kidney beans or mixed beans
¾ cup of oats
2 onions chopped
1 tsp cumin
1 tsp turmeric
1 tsp paprika
½ tsp salt
½ tsp black pepper
Some flour in a dish for dusting
1 tbsp oil for frying

Method

Blitz the onion, beetroot and half the oats together.

Blitz the drained beans and add the oats, beetroot and onion mixture

Add the spices, salt and pepper and stir in well.

Stir in the remaining oats. Mix well and set aside in the fridge for about an hour.

Heat a little oil in a pan.

Get a burger sized amount of the burger mix and dip in the flour. Bring this together in your hands into a burger shape (I wear plastic gloves to stop my hands from turning red...) Dip in flour again until the burger feels firm.

Fry until browned.

You can use whatever spices you like, it's fun to experiment with different mixes.

Note: This mix will make around 12 burgers so you can either halve the ingredients or make a full batch and freeze some for a quick supper.

Leek Lasagne

A delicious pasta free lasagne for you to try.

Ingredients

1 or 2 leeks
½ can chopped tomatoes
8oz ground beef
1 shallot
1 clove garlic
1 tbsp oil
Mozzarella Cheese
Parmesan Cheese
Cottage Cheese

Method

Finely chop the onion and garlic. Heat oil in a pan, add the onions, garlic and ground beef.
Cook for around 5 minutes until the beef is browned.

Add the chopped tomatoes and simmer for 15 minutes.

Cut the leek into 4 inch pieces and open up the leaves to form a flat oblong. Boil in lightly salted water for 2 minutes, strain well and allow to cool.

Layer in small casserole dish as follows:

- Meat sauce,
- Slices of leek (used instead of pasta),
- More meat sauce,
- Spoonful of cottage cheese spread thinly,
- Small pieces of mozzarella. cheese,
- Sprinkling of parmesan cheese.
- Slices of leek,

- Meat sauce,
- Repeat cheeses,
- Then final slices of leek and more cheese.

Bake at 350° until cheese has melted.

Meatloaf Muffins

Ingredients

1 tbsp extra virgin olive oil
300g ground beef
2 minced garlic cloves
1 tsp dried oregano
1 small onion
1 medium zucchini
1 small sweet potato
1 cup tomato paste
⅔ cups flour
Chopped chives

Method

Preheat the oven to 350 °. Grease a 6 hole muffin tin.

Finely chop the onion. Shred the zucchini and sweet potato, squeezing out as much of the excess moisture as you can.

Put all the ingredients except the chives in a large bowl and mix until they're well combined. Don't use all the tomato paste though. You'll need half of the cup for garnishing the meatloaf muffins later.

Spoon the mixture evenly into your muffin tin.

Spread some tomato paste over every beef muffin and sprinkle with chopped chives.

Cook in the oven for 20 minutes at medium heat and serve with a green salad.

Note: If you are making these for a picnic or lunchbox, you could use paper cupcake cases.

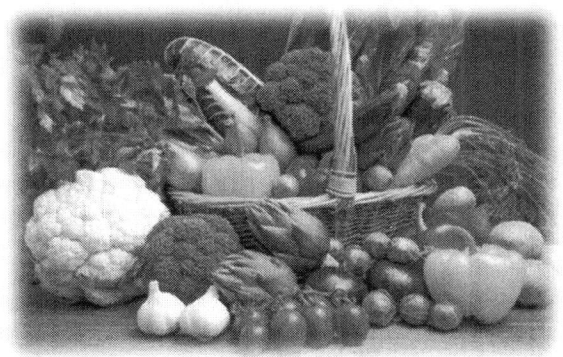

Never underestimate the value of vegetables when thinking about what you are going to make for dinner. They are cheap, delicious and nutritious and can be cooked in many different way.

Also, delicious eaten raw.

Roasted Cauliflower Salad

Ingredients

1 lemon juice
2 tbsp raisins
1 tbsp chill sauce
½ cauliflower
1 red onion
1 tbsp good quality olive oil
1 tsp cumin seeds
½ cup parsley
½ cup cilantro
Sea salt

Method

Preheat the oven to 400° F and prepare a large baking sheet.

In a small bowl, place the raisins, chilli sauce and lemon juice. Whisk all 3 ingredients and set the bowl aside.

Separate the cauliflower head in bite-sized florets using a knife. Slice the onion and finely chop the parsley and cilantro.

Put the florets, onion slices, cumin seeds and oil to the baking sheet. Stir the ingredients with your hands to cover all pieces in oil.

Insert the baking sheet in your oven and leave the veggies to roast for 30 minutes. When the cauliflower florets are light brown remove from the oven and let them cool down.

Transfer everything to a large bowl, including the mixture created from raisins, chilli sauce and lemon juice. Mix all the ingredients using a spoon and season with salt.

Serve immediately with grilled chicken or fish

Mushroom Risotto

This is a very simple recipe and the mushroom can be replaced with anything you happen to have in the fridge. You could add left-over chicken or left-over vegetables or just a handful of herbs.

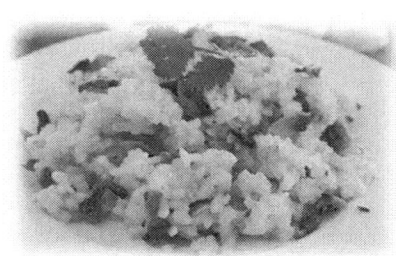

Ingredients

1 tbsp of olive oil
Knob of butter
Small onion
1 clove of garlic
Hot stock (chicken or vegetable)
1 cup Risotto rice
Small handful of frozen garden peas (optional)
Mushrooms – as many as you like
2 tbsp Parmesan cheese
Salt and pepper

Method

Heat the oil and butter in a frying pan and add the onions and garlic. Fry gently until the onion is transparent and soft. Stir in the mushrooms and cook for a few minutes. If using cooked chicken, it will prevent the chicken drying out if you don't add until the rice is almost cooked.

Add the risotto rice and stir until the rice is well combined with the vegetables, butter and oil.

Begin to add the stock, a ladleful at a time, stirring thoroughly. Stir until the stock is absorbed before adding more. Keep adding the stock a ladleful at a time until the rice is soft but with a little bite. The risotto should be creamy.

Add peas if using. Remove from heat and add a tablespoon of parmesan cheese. stir well and season to taste. Sprinkle with the remaining parmesan cheese and serve immediately.

Vegetable Medley Italian Style

The only limit on this dish is your own imagination. This is something I regularly make when I have lots of bits of vegetables left over – usually at the end of the week.

Ingredients

4 large tomatoes
1 small onion
1 clove garlic
1 zucchini
¼ pt vegetable stock
1 tbsp tomato puree
1 tbsp fresh oregano
Seasoning
Parmesan (optional)
1 tbsp toasted flaked almonds
Any other vegetables you have

Method

Skin the tomatoes by putting a cross in the tops of the tomatoes and cover with boiling water. Allow to stand for a minute or two. Remove then plunge into cold water. The skins should be easy to remove. Roughly chop the flesh.

Peel the onion and cut into wedges. Peel and crush the garlic. Slice the zucchini and any other vegetables you have chosen to use.

Heat the stock in a pan then add the garlic, vegetables, tomato puree and fresh herbs. Cover pan and simmer for around 15 minutes until vegetables are tender.

Remove the lid and boil for 4 minutes or until the liquid is reduced and thickened.

Turn out into your serving dish.

Sprinkle the toasted almonds over the vegetables, garnish with a sprinkle of parmesan and some fresh oregano.

Serve immediately.

Zucchini and Cheese Frittata

I love these; I always make one more than I need because I just *know* I'll eat one right away!

Ingredients

1 zucchini
Grated zest of 1 lemon
2 scallions (spring onions)
1 clove garlic
2 tbsp cheddar cheese
1 egg
3 tbsp plain flour
Vegetable oil to shallow fry
Seasoning

Method

Grate the zucchini into a bowl, finely chop the scallions and add the lemon zest, garlic, and cheese. Mix in the egg and stir everything together well.

Gradually add the flour mixing all the time. Just use enough to make the mixture into a thick batter. Season with salt and pepper.

Heat the oil in a frying pan over a medium heat. Carefully drop spoonfuls of the mixture into the oil leaving space between them. Fry over a medium heat for around 3 minutes each side or until nicely golden brown.

Drain on kitchen paper and serve with minted new potatoes and a chili sauce.

Notes:

Cauliflower "Rice" Chicken Stir-Fry

Apart from the cauliflower, the other ingredients in this recipe are optional. You can swap the chicken for prawns and use up any leftover vegetables you have in the refrigerator.

Ingredients

1 cup cauliflower florets
1 chicken fillet
1 tablespoon coconut oil
½ sliced red onion
2 minced cloves garlic
3 tablespoons vegetable stock
½ tablespoon fresh ginger minced
½ small red chili, thinly sliced
1 cup broccoli florets
1 medium carrot, cut into thin strips
½ red bell pepper, stemmed, seeded and diced (optional)
Juice of ¼ lemon
Salt and pepper

Garnish (optional)
1 tbsp shelled pumpkin seeds
1 tbsp fresh cilantro leaves

Method

Place the cauliflower in a food processor and process until it is finely chopped. Add ½ tablespoon coconut oil to a large griddle and set over medium heat. Add ¼ sliced red onion and 1 minced clove garlic and sauté about 4-5 minutes until softened. Stir in the cauliflower and season to taste.

Pour in the vegetable stock, cover with a lid and let cook until all the liquid has evaporated and the cauliflower becomes soft, 5-7 minutes. Remove from the pan and keep covered to stay warm.

In the same pan, heat 1 tablespoon oil over medium heat. Chop the chicken into thin strips and add to pan. Add the remaining red onion and sauté, stirring frequently, until it is golden and translucent. Stir in the remaining garlic, chili and ginger. Cook for 1 minute. Add the bell pepper, carrot and broccoli florets, and sauté stirring frequently until vegetables have softened, 5 minutes. Add the lemon juice, season with salt and turn off the heat.

Place the cauliflower "rice" into a serving plate and top with the roasted vegetables.

Garnish with cilantro and pumpkin seeds. Serve immediately.

Eggs in Bacon Baskets

These little breakfast treats are as delicious as they are impressive and simple to make. They would also make a great lunch served with a nice salad.

Ingredients

4 slices of bacon
1 egg
1 tbsp milk
¼ cup ricotta cheese
Finely chopped parsley (or any herb you prefer)
Chopped chives for garnish
Salt and pepper to taste

Method

Preheat the oven to 350^0F

I use ceramic oven-proof ramekins for this, but if you don't have any, you can use 2 compartments of a muffin pan.

Line 2 ramekins (or muffin pan sections) completely with bacon slices. It works best if you weave the slices. Cut the bacon strips in half if needed to completely cover the bottom and sides of the ramekins. Place in oven for about 5 minutes to start the bacon cooking.

In a measuring cup, break the egg, add the ricotta cheese, milk, salt, pepper, and parsley and whisk until the mixture is evenly mixed. Pour the egg mixture onto the bacon in the ramekins. Put back in oven and bake for 12-15 minutes.

Using a rubber spatula, gently remove the baskets from the ramekin and place on a plate. Sprinkle finely chopped chives over whilst still hot

Serve with hot, buttered toast or, if for a lunch dish, a tomato salad.

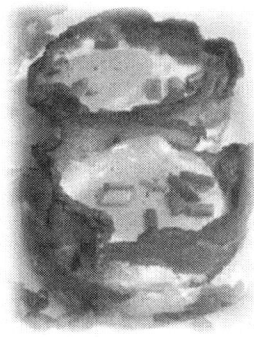

An alternative would be to simply wrap 1 slice of bacon around the outside of a greased ramekin, place in oven for 5 minutes as before, then break a whole egg into the middle and bake until egg is cooked.

Sprinkle with chives when cool.

Note: For a spicy dish you could whisk a bit of chili powder into the egg mixture before pouring into the ramekins.

Garlic and Lemon Beef Tips with Cauliflower Rice

The secret to this dish is that the beef must be cooked very quickly, so that it doesn't have a chance to get tough. This is done all on high heat, and cooks in just 10 minutes. Not strictly a budget dish but I had to include it – it's delicious.

Ingredients

1 small sirloin steak, cut into strips
½ cup beef stock
½ cup white wine
½ cup All-Purpose flour
1 tbsp fresh chopped parsley
1 tbsp olive oil
1 knob of butter
3 tsp chopped garlic
Juice and zest from ½ lemon
1 tsp Onion Powder
Salt and pepper to taste
1 cup cooked cauliflower rice (see *Cauliflower 'Rice' Chicken Stir-Fry* for method)

Method

Cut the sirloin into even sized strips. Add salt and pepper directly to the meat, then toss with the flour until well coated.

Heat olive oil in a non-stick skillet, over high heat. When oil is hot, add the steak, separating each individual strip so that all pieces will brown on all sides. When brown, add garlic and continue cooking for a few seconds. Add the butter. Stir constantly until the butter is melted.

Add the white wine. Continue cooking, stirring occasionally, until the liquid reduces by half. Add the beef stock and stir. Continue cooking until the liquid reduces by half. Add the lemon juice and the zest. Add onion powder, and salt and pepper to taste. Add the parsley. Simmer for just a few more minutes, then turn off the heat.

Make sure your cauliflower rice is warmed through. Serve beef tips over the cauliflower rice, and enjoy.

Baked Vegetable Stuffed Eggplant

The only limit for the stuffing for your eggplant is your imagination. You can mix cheese with the cooked flesh, Cook some bacon and mix that with the flesh etc, etc.

Ingredients

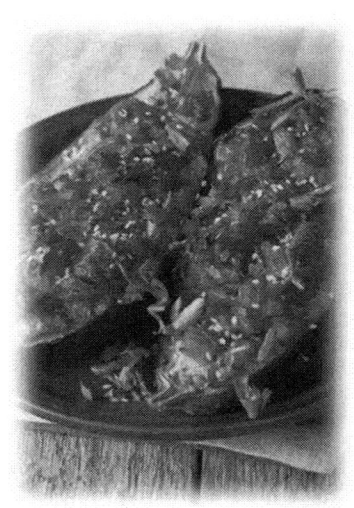

1 eggplant (Aubergine)
2 large tomatoes
1 small onion
1 pepper
1 tbsp olive oil
Chopped cilantro (coriander)
Salt and pepper to taste

Method

Preheat oven to 350° F.

Cut eggplant in half lengthways and place on greased ovenproof tray. Brush both sides with olive oil, season with salt and pepper and bake in oven until eggplant is soft. Remove from oven and scoop out the flesh. Replace outer skin in oven for 5 minutes to crisp up a little.

Meanwhile, chop tomatoes, peppers and onion and fry in a little oil until soft. Mix with some of the eggplant flesh (as much or as little as you like), stir in some chopped cilantro, then fill the skins with the mixture.

Garnish with more chopped cilantro and serve immediately.

Baked Fish in Foil

Ingredients

1 white fish fillet – whichever fish you like best
½ tbsp olive oil
1 fresh jalapeno pepper, chopped (optional)
1 tsp ground black pepper
2 tsps garlic salt
1 lemon, sliced

Method

Preheat oven to 400° F. Wash the fish in the cold water, and pat dry.

Brush the fillet with olive oil, and then sprinkle with black pepper and garlic salt.

Take a large sheet of aluminum foil and place the fillet in the center of it. Place the jalapeno slices on the top, followed by the lemon slices.

Now fold the foil edges over until it resembles an enclosed packet.

Lay the packet onto a baking dish and bake in the oven for 10-15 minutes or until the fish flakes easily with a fork.

Serve with buttered new potatoes and green vegetables. Be careful when opening your foil packet as the steam is very hot!

Note: If you are omitting the jalapeno pepper, you could add a bunch of fresh herbs to add flavor. Fish goes well with basil, chives, marjoram, parsley etc. Even a mix of spices to sprinkle over works well too. Experiment with different flavors until you find your favorite.

Speedy Chicken Chili

I don't know about you but I think any chili tastes so much better the day after. So, I usually make this, leave it in the refrigerator overnight. I reheat thoroughly and have it for dinner the next day usually over a jacket potato – delicious! For me this recipe makes two meals so I freeze some in a foil container but that all depends on your appetite.

Ingredients

1 boneless skinless chicken breast (or any fish or meat you prefer)
½ tbsp vegetable oil
1 small onion, chopped
1 chopped sweet green pepper
1 tsp chili powder
1 tsp dried oregano
½ tsp salt
¼ tsp pepper
½ can diced tomatoes
½ can black beans or kidney beans, drained and rinsed

Method

Trim any fat from chicken breast; cut into small even sized cubes. In large heavy saucepan, heat oil over medium-high heat; cook chicken for about 2 minutes each side or until no longer pink inside. Transfer to plate.

Add onion, green pepper, chili powder, oregano, salt and pepper to pan; cook over medium heat stirring often, for about 5 minutes or until vegetables are softened.

Add tomatoes and beans. Turn up the heat and boil stirring all the time, for 5 around minutes. Put the cooked chicken (or whatever cooked meat or fish you are using) into the sauce and continue to simmer for a further 2 or 3 minutes.

Serve over rice or on its own with chunks of garlic bread.

Note: It is entirely up to you how hot you want your chili, add more or less chili powder according to your own personal taste.

Barbeque Chicken

Delicious served hot or cold so these are a good addition to a packed lunch.

Ingredients

2 chicken drumsticks without skin
1 shallot
1 garlic clove, minced
1 tbsp tomato puree
¼ pint water
2 tbsps red wine vinegar
1 tbsp Worcestershire sauce
1 tbsp mustard

Method

Finely chop the shallot and place in bowl. Add minced garlic, tomato puree, water, vinegar, mustard and Worcestershire sauce. Whisk until well blended.

Rinse the chicken and pat dry with kitchen paper. Place the chicken in an ovenproof dish and pour over the sauce. Leave to stand for at least 2 hours occasionally spooning the sauce over the chicken.

Preheat the oven to 375°F. Cook the chicken in the oven for 20 – 25 minutes or until the juices run clear when a skewer is inserted into the thickest part of the meat.

During cooking spoon the sauce over the chicken a few times to keep moist.

Serve immediately with a few buttered new potatoes or leave to cool and chill in the refrigerator until ready to eat.

Sweet Potato and Tuna Burgers

Ingredients

1 small can tuna in springwater – drained
2 small sweet potatoes
4 spring onions
Handful frozen peas
½ lemon or lime (your choice)
1 egg
3 tbsp oats
Chopped cilantro (optional)
1 tbsp oil

Method

Peel and chop the sweet potatoes into chinks and boil until soft. Finely chop the spring onions. Lightly beat the egg.

Drain the potatoes, place in bowl then mash. Add the tuna, chopped spring onions, frozen peas and mix well. Add the cilantro, zest from lemon and the beaten egg. Mix until everything is combined but not too sticky (you may not need all the egg mix).

Blitz the oats in a blender then place on a flat plate.

Heat the oil in a non-stick pan.

Shape the tuna mix into burger shapes (should make about 4) then cover in the blitzed oats and fry over a medium heat for about 5 minutes each side.

Place onto kitchen paper to drain and serve with a crisp green salad.

Note: I usually have two for dinner and freeze the other two. As I use a full can of tuna I can't make less with this recipe so it could be an ideal dish for when you have a visitor.

Bacon and Chickpea Chunky Soup

Ingredients

4 rashers smoked bacon
½ can drained chickpeas
1 can chopped tomatoes
1 tbsp chopped fresh herbs of your choice or half the amount of dried
2 tsp olive oil
1 cup water
Handful fresh spinach

Method

Put olive oil into pan and fry bacon until cooked.

Add the chickpeas, tomatoes and, if using dried herbs, add these too. If using fresh herbs leave until near the end of cooking.

Pour in 1 cup water. Cover and simmer for around 10 minutes over a low heat.

Remove from heat, stir in the spinach (and fresh herbs if using), cover the pan and leave for 1 minute until spinach is wilted.

Serve and enjoy.

Notes:

Rocket and Avocado Salad with Pine Nuts

Ingredients

2 cups rinsed and dried Rocket (Arugula)
4 cherry tomatoes – halved
¼ cup pine nuts
1 tbsp extra virgin olive oil
¼ tbsp. rice vinegar
¼ cup grated parmesan cheese
1 avocado
1 tbsp lemon juice
Salt and pepper to taste

Method

Whisk together olive oil, rice vinegar, lemon juice and seasoning (for a bit of extra bite you could add half a tsp of chili flakes).

Peel, pit and dice the avocado in a large bowl, add rocket, cherry tomatoes, pine nuts and half the parmesan cheese. Mix together well then dress with the olive oil mixture.

Toss gently then sprinkle with the remaining parmesan cheese.

This is a delicious, summer salad ideal for a lunch box.

Mediterranean Sunday Brunch

Ingredients

1 medium cooked potato
1 tbsp diced pepper
2 or 3 sliced black olives
1 tbsp chopped parsley
2 eggs
¼ tbsp. olive oil
Salt and pepper to taste
2 tbsp ricotta cheese
1 tbsp grated parmesan cheese

Method

Heat a frying pan over a medium high heat and add the olive oil.

Slice the cooked potato thinly and fry gently until golden brown. add the peppers and the black olives and cook until the peppers are soft.

Meanwhile, whisk the eggs, chopped parsley, seasoning and ricotta cheese together well. Pour the mixture over the potatoes and stir together.

Allow the eggs to set but only until still soft on top.

Sprinkle with parmesan cheese and serve immediately.

Sautéed Shrimp, Fennel and Tomatoes

This is a fantastic, fresh dish that is lovely to have at lunchtime with a glass of crisp white wine.

Ingredients

1 tbsp olive oil
1 cup fennel cut into strips
½ can chopped tomatoes
½ tbsp. fresh chopped oregano
1 cup peeled and deveined shrimps
½ cup feta cheese

Method

Heat the o l in a skillet over a medium heat.

Toss in the fennel strips and cook for around 5 minutes or until golden brown. Stir occasionally to stop it catching.

Add the tomatoes and basil and cook for a further 10 minutes adding water if the pan becomes too dry.

Add the shrimps and cook for 2 or 3 minutes until the shrimps are cooked through.

Season to taste and turn out onto serving plate. Crumble the feta cheese over and eat immediately.

Harissa Chicken with Herby Quinoa

Ingredients

1 boneless, skinless chicken breast
1 tsp harissa paste
½ tsp dried oregano
1 tsp olive oil
2 or 3 cherry tomatoes - halved
A few black olives - chopped
½ cup quinoa
Fresh parsley – chopped
Fresh cilantro – chopped (coriander)
Fresh mint – chopped
2 tbsp lemon juice

Method

Mix together the harissa paste and dried oregano. Rub all over the chicken breast and place in a small roasting tin. Leave to marinate for an hour or more.

Preheat oven to 400°F and roast the chicken for 10 minutes. Remove the foil and add the tomatoes and olives.

Return to oven and cook for a further 10 minutes or until the chicken is cooked through.

Meanwhile, cook the quinoa in water according to the packet instructions, then drain and stir in the chopped herbs and lemon juice.

Slice the chicken and place on top of the quinoa then spoon over the tomatoes, olives and any juices from the roasting pan.

Spanish Mackerel with Leek

Mackerel is one of the richest sources of Omega-3 fatty acids and extremely tasty too.

Ingredients

1 mackerel – ask your fishmonger to fillet it for you.
1 tbsp good oil
1 tbsp butter
1 leek
1 tsp paprika
1 tsp dried parsley
1 tsp ground cilantro (coriander)
½ lemon
Salt & pepper to taste

Method

Put paprika, parsley and ground cilantro in a bowl and add a little oil. Mix to form a paste.

Rub each of the fillets with the paste, place in a lightly oiled pan and set aside for about an hour. Preheat the oven to 350°F.

Cover the pan with foil and bake the mackerel for around 10 minutes or until the fish flakes.

Meanwhile, chop the leek into about 1 inch rounds, melt the butter in a pan over a medium heat and add the chopped leeks. Cook for around 10 minutes until soft. Season to taste then arrange on your serving dish.

Top with the mackerel fillets, season to taste and serve with the lemon on the side.

Note: Delicious with a side of deep fried seaweed or just a few boiled potatoes and fresh garden peas.

Spiced Yogurt Chicken

Ingredients

1 boneless skinless chicken breast
2 tbsp natural yoghurt
1 tbsp lemon juice
1 garlic clove – crushed
1 tsp chili flakes
½ tsp paprika
½ turmeric
½ tsp garam masala
2 scallions (spring onion)
Large handful of spinach
1 tbsp chopped fresh cilantro
1 tbsp toasted, flaked almonds
1 tbsp olive oil

Method

Mix together the yogurt, lemon juice, garlic, chili flakes, paprika, turmeric and garam masala with ½ the oil.

Make a few slits in the chicken and cover with the spice mixture. Rub well into the chicken and place in refrigerator for at least 1 hour to marinate.

Preheat the oven to 400°F. Place the chicken in a baking tray, cover with foil and bake for around 30 minutes or until chicken is cooked through.

Meanwhile, heat the remaining oil in a pan, chop the scallions and sauté for 3-4 minutes until softened. Then toss in the spinach and stir until wilted. Season with lots of freshly ground black pepper.

Arrange the spinach on your serving plate, place the chicken breast on top and sprinkle with chopped cilantro and toasted almonds.

Butternut Squash and Goats Cheese Bake

Ingredients

1 small butternut squash
1 sweet potato
1 small red onion
2 tsp fennel seeds
1 tbsp olive oil
1 small goats cheese
Salt and pepper
Chopped rosemary to garnish

Method

Preheat the oven to 400°F.

Peel and deseed the butternut squash and peel the sweet potato and the onion.

Chop all the vegetables into bite sized pieces, mix together well and place into a roasting dish.

Drizzle with olive oil and sprinkle with the fennel seeds then season with salt and pepper.

Roast in the oven for around 20-25 minutes, turning once, until the vegetables are soft and browned.

Cut the goats cheese into chunks and sprinkle over the top of the vegetables. Put back in the oven until the cheese is just beginning to melt – about 5 minutes.

Drizzle with a little olive oil and sprinkle the chopped rosemary over then serve immediately.

Peppered Beef with Sweet Potato Cakes

Ingredients

2 tbsp balsamic vinegar
2 tsp cracked black pepper
1 small rump steak
1 large sweet potato
1 egg
1 tbsp flour
2 tbsp parmesan cheese
1 tbsp olive oil
Large handful rocket (arugula) leaves

Method

Put the balsamic vinegar in a small pan and bubble until it turns syrupy. Set aside.

Put the cracked black pepper on a board and press the steak into t on both sides. Heat a griddle pan and cook the steak for around 2-3 minutes on each side, depending on how you like your steak. Leave to rest for 5 minutes then cut into a few thick slices.

Meanwhile, peel and grate the sweet potato then mix with the egg (beaten) and the flour. Heat the oil in a skillet and drop spoonfuls of the mixture into the pan, flattening slightly with a spatula. Cook for around 3 minutes on each side until cooked and golden. Remove from pan onto kitchen paper.

Arrange salad leaves on your serving plate then top with the sweet potato cakes and peppered beef slices. Drizzle the balsamic glaze over, then serve immediately.

Lamb with Pea and Rosemary Mash

Ingredients

1 large potato suitable for mashing
Large handful frozen or fresh peas
2 tsp chopped rosemary
2 lamb cutlets
2 tsp butter
Salt and pepper to taste

Method

Peel and cook the potatoes in boiling water until tender, adding the peas just before the cooking is finished.

Meanwhile, sprinkle 1 tsp of rosemary over the lamb cutlets and cook on a hot griddle for 2-3 minutes on each side, depending how pink you like your lamb.

Drain the potatoes and peas, return to the pan and lightly mash with the remaining rosemary and the butter. Add salt and pepper to taste then serve with the lamb cutlets on a warmed plate.

Thank You

Thank you for buying this book.

I hope it will help you to eliminate any added sugar from your diet and encourage you to cook fresh food from scratch. In most cases, it doesn't take much longer than putting together a meal full of processed foods – you just need to plan your shopping.

I usually write a list detailing each days food and do my weekly shop just after a meal. You are much less likely to buy 'extras' if you aren't hungry.

Please remember to look carefully at the label of any packaged ingredients you buy. What you think is sugar free can, quite often, have more than you think.

Also, as I said in the introduction, some fresh foods contain naturally occurring sugar so please do your own research.

My next book will be 'Sugar Free Desserts for One' so please keep a look out for it on Amazon.

Good luck on your journey to a Sugar Free life.

Regards

Penny. X

Measurement Conversions

The United States often uses a different measurement system than the rest of the world. There are different units and systems of measurement for different parts of the world, so I've included a few conversions that may help you.

U.S. to metric conversions:

Quantity

1 ounce (fluid) = 29.574 milliliter
1 cup = 236.58 milliliters, or .236 liters, 140 grams (dry)
1 pint = .47 liters
1 quart = .946 liters
1 gallon = 3.785 liters

Weight

1 ounce = 28.35 grams
1 pound = 453.59 grams, or .453 kilograms

Temperature

32°Fahrenheit = 0°Celsius

250°F = Gas mark 1 & 130°C
300°F = Gas mark 2 & 150°C
325°F = Gas mark 3 & 170°C
350°F = Gas mark 4 & 180°C
375°F = Gas mark 5 & 190°C
400°F = Gas mark 6 & 200°C
425°F = Gas mark 7 & 220°C
450°F = Gas mark 8 & 230°C
475°F = Gas mark 9 & 240°C
N.B. If you have a fan oven, the temperature should be reduced by 20°C

Here are some other useful measurement conversions:

1 Cup is equal to:

½ pint
8 ounces
16 Tablespoon
48 Teaspoons
237 milliliters

1 Tablespoon is equal to:

1/16 cup
½ ounce
3 Teaspoons
15 milliliters

1 pint is equal to 2 cups, or .47 liters
1 quart is equal to 4 cups, or .946 liters
1 gallon is equal to 4 quarts, or 16 cups, or 3.79 liters

Convenient Conversions:

¼ cup is equal to 4 Tablespoons, or 2 ounces, or 59 milliliters
½ cup is equal to 8 Tablespoons, or 4 ounces, or 118 milliliters

Family Recipes

Family Recipes

Printed in Poland
by Amazon Fulfillment
Poland Sp. z o.o., Wrocław